Ultimate Anti-aging "What to buy on Amazon" Bible

Your only 100% science based source

by M.K. Arslan, MSc, Mba

Dear Reader,

This single book you are about to read is one of the best investments you can do with your life whether you are an intensely knowledgeable health nut or just a beginner searching for the fountain of youth. This source itself, every action step & every product suggested are based on the latest scientific studies which are listed at the end of the book briefly (links may be subject to change).

To be able to keep this source away from clichés and not useful technical-non technical information, only necessary sentences have been constructed based on methodology for your highly respectful anti- aging attempts. That's why this is the single most concentrated and scientific practical tool in all of your anti-aging attempts. Every single product suggested is specifically chosen on Amazon.com website and ALMOST all the products and brands regarding the interest fields on the website have been investigated carefully for your convenience.

This ebook is written by me who is a life long youth and beauty seeker and spent tremendous amounts of time and efforts in university research labs, projects, scientific literature and cosmetic skincare businesses. That's why in addition to this book's being based on scientific sources, you are 100% at the safe& effective side.

Wishing you a very enjoyable and full of health, happy hours in your beauty seeking awesome journey

Best Regards

Mehmet Kılıç ARSLAN
Chemical Engineer BS, Molecular Biology &Geneticist MSc, Executive MBA

TABLE OF CONTENTS

PROPER SUNSCREEN USAGE AND PREVENTING OTHER SOLAR SIDE EFFECTS

Sunscreen usage

According to the latest science, you had better not use anything other than non-nano zinc oxide based sunscreens for covering wide spectrum (290-400 nm) UVA-UVB protection. 20%-25% ZnO concentrations are fairly enough. You can use zinc oxide based BB-CC creams instead of sunscreen if the ghostly face is your concern.

Suggested products from Amazon;

Badger unscented sunscreen   (Other sunscreens from Badger also ok)

Trukid sunscreen   (Sport one is also ok)

Babo botanicals sunscreen

Loving naturals sunscreen

Juice Beauty sunscreen

Raw Elements sunscreen

For tinted (leaving no white cast) sunscreen I don't advice any mineral powder form. But you can safely use ;

Andalou Naturals BB Cream

Andalou Naturals CC Cream

Juice Beauty CC Cream

Extra Tip *You can even use white color sunscreen from the list above first then a few minutes later put the Andalou BB or CC cream for added protection. No ghostly look, guaranteed.*

Protective clothing

Protective clothing is equally important if not more than sunscreen. Here the most important step towards meeting your high quality expectations is using an UPF sun hat. It has to have at least 3 inch brim in all directions. Another important aspect is, during the hours sunlight does not hit the earth with 90^0 angle, (say 8 to 12 & 2 to 5 pm) hats lose some of their protective functions since light can still kiss your face in a horizontal way. For that issue it's also important for the brim of the hat to be a little bit "bendable" to protect more of your face once needed.

Some protective hat suggestions are;

Tilley airflow hat Probably most stylish look. (Other men-women Tilley hats with at least 3 inch brim can also be used)

Coolibar sun hat (Other men-women Coolibar hats with at least 3 inch brim can also be used)

Columbia sun hat (Other men-women Columbia hats with at least 3 inch brim can also be used)

Physician Endorsed hat (Other women Physician Endorsed hats with at least 3 inch brim can also be used)

Outdoor Research hat (Other men-women Outdoor Research hats with at least 3 inch brim can also be used)

Siggi Bucket hat (Other men-women Siggi Bucket hats with at least 3 inch brim can also be used)

For body clothing, I don't recommend something specifically (shirt, t-shirt, trousers) since it will be very unlikely to wear the same thing outside the house all the time. So, a sun jacket is highly recommended from my own observation.

Coolibar UPF jackets (men/women)

Columbia sportswear women's trail Upf 30

ExOfficio Women's Sol Cool Hooded Zippy Shirt

Driving gloves (you can never know);

Kenmont Summer 100% Cotton Outdoor Sun Uv Protection

Sun umbrella;

Niello ultralight sun umbrella

Yadacme sun umbrella

Lohome UPF umbrella

For sunglasses; It is impossible to suggest anything here since literally thousands of them which equally beneficial are present on the market. Just make sure what you have is 99.9% UVA+UVB protective and big enough to protect your delicate eye area even from the sides. One more thing, make sure it's stylish too.

Indoor lighting

This is also another important missing point to consider in daily life which works cumulatively against your anti aging efforts. Short and simple recipe; change all of the lamps in your house (incandescent, fluorescent, halogen), garage and your working area (hopefully you are good with your boss) with LED lambs. Anything other than certain LED lamps emits UV wavelength. In addition to that, when you go with the LEDs, do not forget to buy them around 2700 K color temperature. Unfortunately anything bigger than 3000-3500 K values will emit some of the unwanted UV spectrum.

Recommendations;

GE Lighting 30915 LED 17-Watt (100-watt replacement)

Solray 6 Pack of LED A19 - 60 Watt Equivalent Soft White (2700K)

Extra Tip *Use blue light filtering application for your phone/tablet/Pc, 7/24*

Sun protective film for home and car windows (for more advanced users)

Gila UV film (99%)

3M Ultra Clear UV protection film

SCIENTIFIC SKINCARE COSMETICS USAGE &ROUTINE

Assuming your only concern is having a healthy skin and preventing& delaying the effects of aging on your face as humanly as possible, in other words you don't have any conditions such as seborrhoeic dermatitis, atopic dermatitis or chronic acne which require a visit to your dermatologist, the best and most scientific skincare anti-aging routine for you basically consists of;

Proper cleansing, using effective serums, moisturizing eye& face, protection (sunscreen or BB/CC creams)

Cleansers

For a good cleanser recommendations;

Burt's Bees Radiance Facial Cleanser

Desert Essence Thoroughly Clean Face Wash Refill

MyChelle Dermaceuticals Creamy Pumpkin Cleanser for Dry Skin

Andalou Naturals 1000 Roses Cleansing Sensitive Foam

Acure Organics Natural Sensitive Face Wash Cleanser With Argan Oil

Island Rx Therapeutic Foaming Facial Cleanser

Mad Hippie Cream Cleanser

Serums

Based on scientific researches there are basically three types of serums you should use that will crown your anti-aging efforts.

I) Vitamin A serum

It can be one of the Vitamin A derivatives including Retinol, Retinoic acid, Retinyl aldehide, Retinyl Retinoate, but stay away from Retynl Palmitate! Another important thing when using Vitamin A serums is always apply them at night. Next day always use sunscreen (as always).

Lastly, depending on the physical characteristics of the serum bottle, try to buy a pumped serum dispenser if possible. In any other circumstances serum exposure to air should have been minimized to prevent oxidized chemicals production. Better keep the serum in fridge and take the necessary amount as fast as possible then seal the bottle tightly. Don't use the Vitamin A serum at the same night when you do exfoliation to your face (AHA, BHA, PHA). I don't advice using it with Vitamin C serum at the same time either.

Amazon shopping guide;

SkinCeuticals Retinol 1.0 Maximum Strength Refining Night Cream

Retinol Cream Moisturizer 2.5% - 3.4 OZ Firming Anti-Aging

Mad Hippie Skin Care Products Vitamin A Serum

Joyal Beauty Retinol Serum for Face by Joyal Beauty

MyChelle Dermaceuticals Remarkable Retinal Serum for Anti-Aging Defense

Beauty Essentials Retinol Serum 2.5% For Fine Lines, Wrinkles, Acne Scars, Dark Spots, Sun Damage

Eve Hansen 2 oz Retinol (Vitamin A) - Facelift in a Bottle

II) Vitamin C serum

Vitamin C serum is one of the biggest investments you can do for your skin besides using sunscreen. You had better stay away from Ascorbyl Palmitate (as in the Retinyl Palmitate) but can safely use l-ascorbic acid, tetrahexyl decyl ascorbate, sodium ascorbyl phosphate and magnesium ascorbyl phosphate options. Serum's exposure to air should be prohibited as strictly as possible if cannot totally be prevented. So an airless pump or an amber color glass is the best possible options to use Vitamin C serum to get the maximum benefit.

Amazon shopping guide;

Mad Hippie Vit C Serum, Anti-oxidant

Azure Naturals - ULTIMATE Vitamin C Serum 22% Advanced Proprietary Blend Vitamin C E Ferulic

Organic Vitamin C Serum 20% for Face by Joyal Beauty

Born In Nature's 20% Vitamin C Facial Serum + E + Vegan Hyaluronic & Ferulic Acid

Skinceuticals C E Ferulic

Truskin Naturals Vitamin C Serum for Face with Hyaluronic Acid, 20% C + E Professional Topical Facial Skin Care

Amara Organics Vitamin C Serum for Face 20% with Hyaluronic Acid & Vitamin E

III) Peptide& Antioxidant serum

Last science based serums which will keep your skin supple and enhance your anti aging success are high quality peptide based and antioxidant serums. Antioxidant serums are strongly advised to be used after Vitamin C serum and just before the sunscreen, while peptide based serums are better used interchangeably at the nights when Vitamin A serum is not used.

Amazon shopping guide;

Peptide based serums;

Mad Hippie Face Cream with Anti Wrinkle Peptide Complex

Visio Elan BEST 3 Peptide Firming Serum With Hyaluronic Acid & Collagen - Lift & Tighten Facial Skin, Neck & Around Eyes

Pronu Peptide Complex Serum - Copper Peptide, Swiss Apple Stem and Argireline

Natural Science Skincare Anti-Aging Moisturizing Skin Cream For Face & Body with Matrixyl 3000 Peptides & Hyaluronic Acid and Vitamin C Serum

Amara Organics Anti Aging Face Cream Moisturizer with Resveratrol & Peptides

Derma e Peptides Plus Double-Action Wrinkle Reverse Serum

Antioxidants based serums for added boost;

Andalou Naturals Fruit Stem Cell Revitalize Serum with Resveratrol Q10

Mad Hippie Antioxidant Facial Oil

Ageless Derma Super Green Moisturizing Serum with Certified Organic Ingredients

Andalou Naturals Tumeric Plus C Enlighten Serum

Moisturizers

Again it's hard to recommend a good facial moisturizer since so many great ones are on the market, still you will be foolproof and at the safe side by choosing one of the listed below that all contain a good moisturizer needs (humectants, emollients, occlusive, cell communicating ingredients, stable chemistry, good price level).

Amazon shopping guide;

Body Merry Anti Aging Night Cream Moisturizer with 5% Niacinamide

Block Island Organics - Organic Revitalizing Night Cream with Antioxidants

Keys Luminos Hydrating Moisturizer

Weleda Age Revitalizing Night Cream

Acure Day Cream Gotu Kola Stem Cell + 1% Chlorella (Use at night!)

Eye "Cream"

Yes you heard it right, it has to have a creamy texture and/or include plenty of occlusive ingredients to be able to prevent unwanted drying effects for this delicate area. Practically a not very viscous eye serum on its own is not enough for the eyes, check for the suggestions below.

Amazon shopping guide;

Beauty without Cruelty Green Tea Nourishing Eye Gel

Amara Organics Eye Cream for Dark Circles and Puffiness with Peptides

Clareye - Eye Cream For Dark Circles, Puffiness, Wrinkles

Dr. Hauschka Daily Hydrating Eye Cream

Truskin Eye Gel Cream for Wrinkles, Fine Lines, Dark Circles, Puffiness

SCIENTIFICALLY PROVEN TECHNOLOGICAL GADGETS FOR YOUR WELL-BEING

Microcurrent, red light therapy or radiofrequency. According to the latest research findings these therapies are not very good investments to buy and try at home on your face to gain significant benefits, let alone the unwanted side effects such as overstimulation of muscles which can create further wrinkles! To begin with, while blue-red lights have some proven advantages on the treatment of skin lesions (such as acne) or on the creation of some collagen fibers, on the other hand their creating more ROS (Reactive oxygen species such as singlet oxygen) while our aim is the complete opposite, it leaves a very big question mark against the usage of this devices on your face. If you are still very keen on using these devices put a strong antioxidants serum on your face first (such as green tea extract). Then use a FDA approved one (such as Baby Quasar).

Radiofrequency devices are also somewhat beneficial about increasing the collagen thickness in dermis, yet they create significant amount of heat and don't have a long history of safety records. So these types of devices may better be used under the supervision of a dermatologist for fixing a problem such as keloids or acne, and better be kept out of the home. Again nothing to buy in Amazon or no Thermage on your face☺

When it comes to microcurrent devices, a clear no, they are not helping you lift your face aka facelift. Not one credible double blinded scientific research there is on the anti-aging profits side but if you have a wound or scar on your face they can probably help the healing process. Ergo, again unnecessary at home, but maybe used in the doctors' office for certain situations.

In addition to those there is a very simple device I can advice for your delicate faces. Foreo Luna (or its derivatives) technically which is not a high tech gadget but may provide some benefits to the user by providing sonic vibrations to enhance the circulation and lymph drainage while increasing the efficiency of facial cleansing gels assuming no one properly cleanse their faces with bare hands although there is not scientific evidences on that. On the other side of the equation ,Clarisonic Mia, I am not saying it's not safe and ineffective but there is no research done that shows it does not create micro tears on your face. Also it makes your skin TOO MUCH clean which is not a very good idea while your skin tries to have a balanced amount of healthy flora. Over exfoliating and damaging stratum corneum are my other concerns but it may still not be that bad of an idea to give it a try for some individuals.

SOLO Mio Sonic Face Cleanser and Massager Brush (No difference in principal with Foreo Luna so you don't have to pay more for the same gains)

PLUSES THAT CAN BE ACHIEVED BY LIFE STYLE IMPROVEMENTS

How to make your own lifesaving lists;

-Try to hit a good 8 hours of sleep. It's proven that adding even as less as 30 minutes more sleep to your regular sleep regimen (6-7 hours) helps you gain substantial benefits. On the other hand, do not sleep more than 9 hours which start to work counterproductive for your metabolism after this threshold.

-While protecting yourself from sunrays as much as possible by using sunscreen and UPF clothing is a very good strategy , actually getting some sun is nevertheless good for you. There are about 30,000 genes in a human chromosome and vitamin D takes part in about 3,000 of their expressions. Here the key part is, it's not very important which parts of your body get the sun since it's converted to its final state 25- OH Vitamin D in the kidneys. So it's wise to go strategically and absorb like 5-10 minutes of sun exposure on your back, back of your legs or bottom area of yours while still protecting your face.

-Sleep on your back- definitely and absolutely. While using satin/silk pillowcases to get rid of the potential friction of the materials on your face, you still need to distribute the gravity evenly and had better not squash your face lying on your front or on your side. Definitely a game changer one! You can try to put a small pillow under your knees if you have a hard time in adaptation at first.

Amazon shopping guide;

Myface Pillow (The best one. If your head is of a larger size you may still use it by removing some of the wings with your hands).

-Use a shower filter. Good for your skin, good for your hair, good for lungs etc..

Amazon shopping guide;

Sprite All Brass High Output Chrome Shower Filter with Matching Chrome Head (NSF certified)

Sprite HO2-WH-M Universal Shower Filter and 3 Setting Shower Head (NSF certified)

AquaBliss High Output Universal Shower Filter with Replaceable 3-Stage Filter

-Use an air purifier. Another though one to pick since so many great models with so many filtering combinations are on the market. Just be careful about the filter medias which are used in your air purifier (carbon, TRUEhepa) have antibacterial coatings. Also be sure that they allow you to turn off their Ionizer functions if they have any. Even if they claim that the amount of ozone off gassed to air is under legal limitations, there are other dangers at least as big as the ozone problem (inhaling ROS& aggregated contaminants). To be on the extra safe side, don't buy unit with UVC either. All in all, just a plain carbon (antibacterial)+TRUEhepa (antibacterial) filters are enough in dealing most of the contaminants. So I won't recommend any $500+ air purifier which may be necessary only if you are under extremely serious threats regarding to the air quality.

Amazon shopping guide;

AeraMax 200 Air Purifier for Allergies and Odors with True HEPA Filter and 4-Stage Purification

PureZone 3-in-1 True HEPA Air Purifier - 3 Speeds Plus UV-C Air Sanitizer (UVC function can be turned off)

For desktop;

Holmes HEPA-Type Desktop Air Purifier with 3 Speeds and Quiet Operation

Bonus Tip: It is a great pleasure for me to introduce you one of the biggest contributions you can do for yourself, which is buying one of these things that are the only kind of their own and can add extreme amounts of benefits to you in the long run. Though they have ionizers that can't be turned off, still benefits far outclass the side effects especially if you are living in a polluted city.

Smart Gadgets 2016 Wearable Air Purifier Negative Ion Generator, HEPA Filter Li-ion Powered Fan (2 Wind Speeds)

SCIENTIFIC ANTI-AGING NUTRITION

This topic is normally a whole encyclopedia on its own so its integral is taken and divided into most easy to use and practical way for the convenience. Since this is not a nutrition or weight loss book, only anti-aging related purchases will be included here. So aside from a balanced diet in which there are lots of alternatives depending on your aims (weight loss, gain muscle, decreasing fat ratio, being vegan etc..) as a general anti-aging approach, the most useful and realistic way to consider will be those which includes using smoothie machines (blender) and juicers beside steam cooking your daily vegetables and whatever you are eating. I personally advice to use portable blenders ,which are easy to clean for the sake of ease, interchangeably with slow juicers to prevent oxidation as much as possible and provide the most amount of juice output.

Amazon shopping guide;

Blender;

Nutri Ninja Pro

Nutribullet Pro Deluxe Edition 900-Watt Smoothie Juice Blender

Personal Blender With Travel Lid - 21oz Portable Sports Bottle

Juicers;

Omega J8006 Nutrition Center Juicer

Kuvings NJE-3580U Masticating Slow Juicer

Panasonic MJ-L500 Slow Juicer with Frozen Treat Attachment

I don't recommend juicing every day, but it's a great way from time to time to get health boosts. You should immediately drink the juice from the juicer to prevent oxidation since the liquid contains virtually no fiber. You can prepare yourself a very healthy drink by using the vegetables you normally don't prefer to eat such as cabbage, broccoli, celery, roman lettuce etc.

When it comes to smoothies, because of their high fiber content it's possible to drink them more slowly throughout the day without much concern unlike it was for the juicing. What I suggest you is to cover as much variety of superfood products as possible which may help you in your anti-aging goals, since most of them is scientifically proven to be valuable in your diet. You can use the following superfoods both raw, in your meals, or as a smoothie ingredients;

Berries (all types of berries especially red grapes with skin and seeds), cruciferous vegetables, pomegranate, avocado, coconut, brazil nuts, chia seeds, quinoa, amaranth, flaxseed (only if you are a woman!), tomato, cocoa powder, walnut, lemon

Also try to consume these as much as possible in your meals;

Turmeric, curry powder, ginger, garlic, onion, rosemary, wild salmon, kefir (milk/coconut), green tea (better white tea), cinnamon, olive oil, bone broth.

USAGE OF ANTIOXIDANTS AND OTHER LIFE ENHANCING METHODS ACCORDING TO THE LATEST SCIENTIFIC DATA

I personally DO NOT recommend the use of any pills or supplements for very long periods of time continuously under normal circumstances, but of course if it is related to your medical condition (age, disease, pregnancy etc.) and given by your family doctor, you have to follow the directives. If you scientifically consider the current cumulative knowledge level about redox reactions as a responsible and knowledgeable scientist, it's hard to claim otherwise I believe. In most of the cases supplements do nothing if not harming you. BUT still there are some important points you should consider if you are aiming to reach your anti aging policies as scientific and economic as possible.

-DO NOT take normal multivitamins (A,B,K, E etc..) under normal conditions. Medical necessity is something different and talk to your MD for details.

-Still you better take some pills actually, especially if you are not consuming a fair amount of omega-3 & Vitamin D sources (especially fishes which are not contaminated with cadmium, mercury and PCBs such as sardines& anchovies).

-If you are still insisted on using "something" it's better to consume green whole food powders which are created using natural whole foods and can also be blended with your daily smoothie.

So the total scheme should be like this;

Organic, raw/steamed real food chewed by your teeth--> Plenty of daily

Smoothie--> Good amount of daily if you are sure it has good amount of vegetables in it

Home Juicing--> Occasionally, 1-2 times a week

Green Powder--> If you are really keen to do something extra. But total waste of money form if you drink smoothie daily

Multivitamins--> Do not! (unless you have been advised under a medical practitioner as mentioned previously)

BUT, when it comes to specialty promising superstars that will add the real boost to your efforts and have already been worked in researches though not completely scientifically fail proof (not having placebo controlled, double blinded, long term human studies in each but still very promising results in current studies), these are basically;

PLE;

Amazon shopping guide;

SunPill UV Skin Support Tabs 30 ct

Heliocare Oral Capsules

Life Extension Enhanced Fernblock with Sendara Mineral Supplements

Glocosamine;

Actif Joint 4-in-1 Fast Relief Maximum Strength, Clinically Proven Formula, 120ct, Made in USA

VISCODERM Pearls 30 softpearls   (Hello UK!)

PQQ;

Jarrow Formulas Ubiquinol Plus Pyrroloquinoline Quinone

Doctor's Best PQQ Nutritional Supplement

Pterostilbene;

Life Extension Pteropure Pterostilbene Vegetarian Capsules, 50 mg, 60 Count

Absorb Health Pterostilbene | 100mg | 100 Capsules

Nicotinamide Riboside

NIAGEN 300 Nicotinamide Riboside (NR), Patented Energy Optimizer

HPN Nutraceuticals NIAGEN

(You can buy Pterostilbene+ Nicotinamide Riboside in the same "Basis" from Elysium.com also)

Vitamin C (Try to hit 1000 mg. Vitamin C daily)

The Organique Co. Organic Raw Camu Camu Superfood Powder

Terrasoul Superfoods Organic Acerola Cherry Powder

Terrasoul Superfoods Amla Powder

Dear reader, I assume we are kinda friends now with the philosophy that people who are sharing the same emotions and walking towards similar targets even thousands of miles away are actually close. I know and I know very well that if you read this book you already know that our journey is a very long one by its nature, but reading this book and applying its principles which are based on pure science , now you are more close to your healthy, beautiful and full of happiness life journey. You may contact me anytime from my personal linked-in page as well as the facebook page you can find with my name.

Yours truly

Mehmet K. Arslan

Sources:

Commonly used UV filter toxicity on biological functions: review of last decade studies

Microfine zinc oxide (Z-Cote) as a photostable UVA/UVB sunblock agent

Microfine Zinc Oxide is a Superior Sunscreen Ingredient to Microfine Titanium Dioxide

DNA damaging potential of zinc oxide nanoparticles in human epidermal cells

-----

On the course of the irritant reaction after irritation with sodium lauryl sulphate

Cleansing Formulations That Respect Skin Barrier Integrity

Detergent-induced epidermal barrier dysfunction and its prevention

Effect of commercial cleansers on skin barrier permeability

Retinyl retinoate induces hyaluronan production and less irritation than other retinoids

Synthesis and in vitro biological activity of retinyl retinoate, a novel hybrid retinoid derivative

Application of l-Ascorbic Acid and its Derivatives (Sodium Ascorbyl Phosphate and Magnesium Ascorbyl Phosphate) in Topical Cosmetic Formulations: Stability Studies

Skin anti-aging strategies

Vitamin C in dermatology

Photoprotective potential of lycopene, β-carotene, vitamin E, vitamin C and carnosic acid in UVA-irradiated human skin fibroblasts

Comparison of clinical efficacies of sodium ascorbyl phosphate, retinol and their combination in acne treatment

-----

Semin Cutan Med Surg. Author manuscript; available in PMC 2014 Aug 8.

Light emitting diode-generated blue light modulates fibrosis characteristics: Fibroblast proliferation, migration speed, and reactive oxygen species generation

A study to determine the efficacy of combination LED light therapy (633 nm and 830 nm) in facial skin rejuvenation

Facial Rejuvenation in the Triangle of ROS. *Crystal Growth & Design*, 2009;

Low-intensity electrical stimulation in wound healing: review of the efficacy of externally applied currents resembling the current of injury.

Air purifiers that diffuse reactive oxygen species potentially cause DNA damage in the lung

-----

Effects of different cooking methods on health-promoting compounds of broccoli

Effects of different cooking methods on the vitamin C content of selected vegetables

USDA Table of Nutrient Retention Factors

Domestic cooking methods affect the nutritional quality of red cabbage

-----

Discovering the link between nutrition and skin aging

Antioxidants and Exercise: More Harm Than Good?

Antioxidants: In Depth

Food and Vitamins and Supplements! Oh My!

The effect of fruit and vegetable powder mix on hypertensive subjects: a pilot study

Polypodium leucotomos as an Adjunct Treatment of Pigmentary Disorders

A comprehensive toxicological safety assessment of an aqueous extract of Polypodium leucotomos (Fernblock®)

Sunscreen in a Pill?

A dietary supplement improves facial photoaging and skin sebum, hydration and tonicity modulating serum fibronectin, neutrophil elastase 2, hyaluronic acid and carbonylated proteins

The effect of an oral supplement containing glucosamine, amino acids, minerals, and antioxidants on cutaneous aging: a preliminary study

Dietary pyrroloquinoline quinone (PQQ) alters indicators of inflammation and mitochondrial-related metabolism in human subjects

Pyrroloquinoline quinone stimulates mitochondrial biogenesis through cAMP response element-binding protein phosphorylation and increased PGC-1alpha expression.

Low-dose pterostilbene, but not resveratrol, is a potent neuromodulator in aging and Alzheimer's disease

A Review of Pterostilbene Antioxidant Activity and Disease Modification

Partial reversal of skeletal muscle aging by restoration of normal NAD$^+$ levels

Inhibition of de novo NAD(+) synthesis by oncogenic URI causes liver tumorigenesis through DNA damage

Advanced glycation end products

www.ingramcontent.com/pod-product-compliance
Lightning Source LLC
Chambersburg PA
CBHW070257290526
45789CB00004B/1884